D0861950

The Fertility Manual

The Fertility Manual

Reproductive Options for Your Family

Dorette Noorhasan, MD

BROWN BOOKS
PUBLISHING GROUP

© 2019 Dorette Noorhasan, MD

All rights reserved. No part of this book may be used or reproduced in any manner without written permission except in the case of brief quotations embodied in critical articles or reviews.

This book is based on the personal experiences of the author. It is not intended to diagnose any condition and is not to be considered a substitute for consultation with a licensed professional. As the study and treatment of infertility is an evolving field in which methods, statistics, and terminology may change in response to new research, always consult your medical team before making any decisions regarding treatment.

The Fertility Manual
Reproductive Options for Your Family

Brown Books Publishing Group
16250 Knoll Trail Drive, Suite 205
Dallas, Texas 75248
www.BrownBooks.com
(972) 381-0009

A New Era in Publishing®

Publisher's Cataloging-In-Publication Data

Names: Noorhasan, Dorette, author.
Title: The fertility manual : reproductive options for your
    family / Dorette Noorhasan, MD.
Description: Dallas, Texas : Brown Books Publishing Group,
    [2019]
Identifiers: ISBN 9781612543284
Subjects: LCSH: Infertility--Popular works. | Infertility-
    -Treatment--Popular works. | Human reproductive
    technology--Popular works. | Pregnancy--
    Complications--Popular works.
Classification: LCC RC889 .N66 2019 | DDC 616.692--dc23

ISBN 978-1-61254-328-4
LCCN 2019939249

Printed in the United States
10 9 8 7 6 5 4 3 2 1

For more information or to contact the author, please go to
www.DrDoretteNoorhasan.com.

To everyone struggling with infertility.

CONTENTS

Introduction

Fertility struggles have always been a part of life; today, however, it seems that infertility is more prevalent than ever. This spike is likely caused by a true increase in infertility due to societal changes combined with a higher awareness of infertility issues. In recent decades, waiting longer to initially conceive, potential exposure to toxic chemicals, and the desire to have children with new partners later in life have all contributed to an increase in individuals and couples seeking reproductive help. As a society, we are gradually becoming more comfortable speaking out about our struggles with fertility. It seems that we all know someone who is struggling to become a parent.

My goal is to educate you about the fertility process so you can ask the right questions that will ultimately benefit you with a successful pregnancy. I will avoid excessive medical jargon and provide you with facts. This book is not meant to be a large reference guide that sits on your desk but a book that you read a few days before seeing the fertility doctor for your first visit. Having personally gone through my own fertility journey to have my son, I understand the patient's perspective. As struggling with infertility can take a huge mental and emotional toll on the participants, the last chapter of this book is dedicated to the psychological aspect of infertility. Ideally, the content of the book should be as accessible as having a conversation with a friend who is knowledgeable on the subject.

This book reflects the latest reproductive treatments currently available. However, fertility is a field of ever-changing technology. The first *in vitro fertilization* (IVF) baby, Louise Brown, was born in 1978. The field of reproductive endocrinology and infertility has come a long way since 1978 and continues to grow. Babies born from frozen sperm, from frozen embryos, or from frozen eggs were once a dream but are now a reality. I look forward to updating this book in a few years as technology evolves.

The content of this book is not intended as medical advice; it is intended as an overview of fertility, improving your understanding of the process so that it is less intimidating and giving you the confidence to ask the right questions as you seek treatment. We are all individuals with unique situations and problems, so I encourage you to seek the care of a medical professional who knows your history and can work with you to achieve parenthood. Having knowledge of key fertility issues will equip you to ask your doctor the right questions, will inform you about what options are available, and will ultimately lead to the best chance of a successful pregnancy. So here we go. Take notes, and enjoy the journey to parenthood.

One

Before You See the Doctor

QUESTION:

How do I know if I should see a doctor about infertility?

ANSWER:

Generally, if you are a woman age thirty-four or younger, have been having unprotected intercourse for twelve months, and haven't gotten pregnant, you should see a physician. If you are thirty-five years of age or older, you should see a doctor after six months of unprotected intercourse. In some situations, you should not wait to see a doctor. These include:

- Blocked *fallopian tubes*, also called *tubal factor*. The fallopian tubes are tubal structures in which the *sperm* and egg unite to form the *embryo* and which are then used to transport the embryo to the *uterus*.
- Lack of ovulation.
- Abnormal sperm, also called *male factor*, as the sperm is the male reproductive cell.

Women at risk for tubal factor include women with a history of prior pelvic inflammatory diseases (such as gonorrhea or chlamydia), prior *ectopic pregnancies* (meaning that the pregnancy implanted outside the uterus), or prior *tubal ligation* (a form of sterilization in which the fallopian tubes are bound, transected, or completely removed). Women who do not ovulate regularly will generally not have regular periods and should see a physician when trying to conceive. Examples of male factor include prior infections, prior testicular diseases, a previous vasectomy, and steroid or testosterone usage. Additionally, you should see a physician to help you conceive if you are in a same-sex relationship or if you are a single man or single woman wanting to have children without a partner. Parenthood is a real possibility for all of us.

QUESTION:

What should I do before I see a fertility physician?

ANSWER:

There are multiple aspects to this question's answer.

1. **Your health:** Women should make sure their Pap smears and mammograms are up to date. If you have chronic medical conditions, you should make sure that these are well-controlled before conceiving. For example, if you have diabetes, you should make sure your sugars are under control first, as abnormal sugars can have a negative impact on a pregnancy. Also, weight can negatively

impact conceiving and can increase a woman's risk for miscarriage. A normal body mass index (BMI) is 18.5–24.9, while a BMI of 25–29.9 is considered overweight. BMIs of 30 and greater are considered obese. If your BMI is high, weight loss can improve your chances of conceiving and carrying to full term. Similarly, women with a very low BMI or low body-fat percentage can also have problems ovulating and, hence, conceiving. Additionally, you should make sure your immunizations are up to date. The measles, mumps, and rubella (MMR) and varicella (chicken pox) vaccines cannot be given during pregnancy, so make sure these are up to date before conceiving. If you smoke, drink excessive alcohol, drink excessive caffeine, or use illicit drugs, you should start cutting back with a goal of completely quitting before conceiving. Women should start a prenatal vitamin, and men should start a multivitamin.

2. **Insurance:** You should contact your insurance company or the human resources department of your employment office. Many insurance plans cover testing for infertility, and some cover treatment. Coverage can vary from company to company and from state to state, so you will want to get a good understanding of your benefits.

3. **Research:** Talk to your obstetrician/gynecologist, and get recommendations on fertility physicians in your

area. Speak with your friends and family. Many of them could know someone who has successfully done fertility treatments in your area. Research various fertility clinics online; however, it is hard to use online reviews as your sole source of recommendations. Always take both the positive and negative reviews with a grain of salt. There might be aspects of that patient's care that are not reflected in their review. I recommend comparing the IVF success rates of different clinics through websites such as the Society for Assisted Reproductive Technology (SART. org) or the Centers for Disease Control and Prevention (CDC.gov), which strive to compare clinics objectively. Keep in mind, though, that these sites receive their data directly from the clinics, which can "cherry-pick" which favorable patients go through IVF and thereby boost their IVF pregnancy rates.

QUESTION:

What should I do before the first appointment with the fertility specialist?

ANSWER:

You should fill out all of your paperwork ahead of time and plan to bring a copy of all your previous records. If possible, send these records ahead of time so the doctor has time to look at them. Although it's not a requirement, you should bring your partner or a friend to the appointment if possible.

The information can be overwhelming, so having a second set of ears in the room will help you make the most of your appointment.

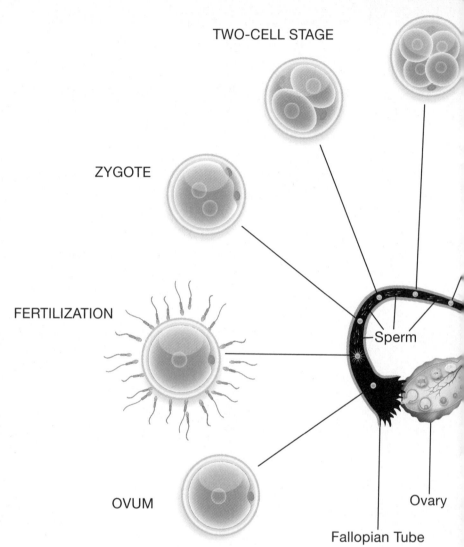

FOUR-CELL STAGE

TWO-CELL STAGE

ZYGOTE

FERTILIZATION

Sperm

OVUM

Ovary

Fallopian Tube

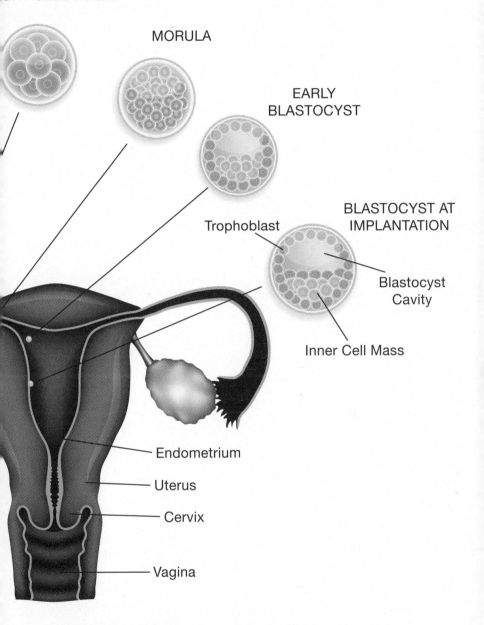

MORULA

EARLY
BLASTOCYST

BLASTOCYST AT
IMPLANTATION

Trophoblast

Blastocyst
Cavity

Inner Cell Mass

Endometrium

Uterus

Cervix

Vagina

Figure 1: Female reproductive tract demonstrating ovulation of the ovum (egg), fertilization of the ovum by sperm, development and migration of the embryo to the uterus, and implantation of the embryo in the uterus.

Two

Your First Visit: Getting a Diagnosis

QUESTION:

What should I expect at my first visit to the fertility doctor?

ANSWER:

Your first visit is very important for numerous reasons. Plan to be there for at least one to two hours. Not all of this time will be spent with the doctor; a large portion of it will be dedicated to meeting the front desk staff, filling out paperwork, and meeting the nurse to review details of the doctor's recommended plan. This is also a good time for you to figure out whether this clinic is the right fit for you.

QUESTION:

Describe the first encounter with the fertility doctor.

ANSWER:

If you have already had testing or treatments at another location, the doctor will review your records and make further recommendations. If you are new to the fertility world, your doctor will educate you regarding several tests that need to be done before treatment can be recommended. The list of tests can be rather long, but there are good reasons to do extensive testing before making treatment recommendations. Your doctor needs to identify the problem (or problems) in order to determine the best treatment for you. Most problems with conception are tied to abnormalities either in the structure of reproductive organs or in their function. This is what the testing will help identify.

Four major categories of the reproductive system need to be evaluated. Additionally, the psychological aspect should be evaluated as well.

1. Eggs

Eggs (*oocytes*) need to be of both good quantity and good quality. The quantity and quality of eggs is called *ovarian reserve*. The more advanced a woman's age, the lower her ovarian reserve. Ovarian reserve generally is good in our twenties and starts to decrease in our thirties, with steeper decreases in our forties. Typically, by the time a woman is in her midforties, she has an incredibly low chance of conceiving with her own eggs and will require donor eggs, if she chooses. Remember, however, that we are all different. I have provided the general population's characteristics based on age, but we are all individuals. There are women in their twenties who may also need donor eggs and women in their forties who will conceive easily.

Your doctor will do a sonogram (ultrasound) to look at your ovaries and uterus. The sonogram will give an estimate of the *antral follicle count* (AFC). *Follicles* are the houses of the eggs within the ovaries. AFC is the number of follicles in both ovaries at any given point in time. A normal AFC is approximately eight to ten but declines with age. Therefore, it is normal to see an AFC of four in a forty-year-old woman. AFC can be excessively high in women who do not ovulate, such as those with *polycystic ovarian syndrome* (PCOS).

Your doctor will also order many blood tests to get an idea of your ovarian reserve. *Follicle stimulating hormone* (FSH) and *estradiol* (E2) are hormonal blood tests typically drawn on the second, third, or fourth day of the menstrual cycle. The E2 level must always be drawn with the FSH; otherwise, the FSH is uninterpretable. An FSH under 10 mIU/L with a low E2 level suggests a good ovarian reserve. An FSH of greater than 10 mIU/L is considered abnormal, and FSH values greater than 20 mIU/L suggest very low chances of conceiving using your own eggs. FSH values, however, vary from cycle to cycle. In some menstrual cycles, the value may be normal, and in others, it may be abnormal. The key is to look for a consistent pattern. An *anti-Mullerian hormone* (AMH) test is another hormonal blood test for ovarian reserve. AMH is produced by the granulosa cells of the ovarian follicle. The higher the AMH value, the more suggestive of a higher quantity of remaining eggs. Unlike FSH, AMH is more consistent from menstrual cycle to menstrual cycle. Generally, AMH declines with age, and it can be slightly suppressed when on an oral contraceptive pill (OCP) or when breastfeeding. Even though there is a widespread belief that AMH can be drawn at any point in the menstrual cycle, many studies now suggest that AMH is best drawn in the *follicular phase*.[1] Additionally, there are several *assays* (ways to analyze AMH values), with some variability between assays. Therefore, an AMH drawn at one lab can be different from an AMH drawn at another lab.

In addition to having good ovarian reserve, you need to ovulate (release an egg) to conceive. Often, fertility specialists do not test for ovulation because we will give you medications to make your body ovulate. The following is a brief description of the menstrual cycle and ovulation.

The menstrual cycle typically lasts twenty-eight days, with a normal range of twenty-one to thirty-five days.[2] Cycle day 1 (CD 1) is the first day of full flow of menses. If you spot for several days before your period starts, do not count the days of spotting; the first day of full flow is considered CD 1. After that point, you begin to count the days: CD 1, CD 2, CD 3, etc., until CD 28 (or the last day of the cycle), and then CD 1 of the next cycle. In a twenty-eight-day cycle, women will generally ovulate around CD 14, as ovulation typically happens fourteen days before the onset of the next period. Therefore, a woman with a thirty-day cycle will ovulate around CD 16. The first half of the menstrual cycle (from CD 1 to ovulation) is called the follicular phase. The second half of the menstrual cycle (from ovulation to the next menses) is called the *luteal phase*. *Progesterone* is a hormone that becomes elevated after ovulation. Typically, progesterone level is measured about seven days after ovulation (and therefore about seven days before the next menses). This is a called the *midluteal phase* and is the time at which progesterone is usually at its highest value for that menstrual cycle. If you do not have regular menstrual cycles, then chances are you are not ovulating. However, occasionally, a woman with "regular" cycles might not ovulate, and a woman with "irregular" cycles might ovulate once in a while.

2. Sperm

Sperm also need to be of good quantity and quality. The basic test for evaluating this is a semen analysis, which assesses many parameters. Generally, men are asked to spend two to five days in abstinence prior to producing the sample for the semen analysis, although some clinics will allow two to seven days of abstinence. Less than two days results in a smaller volume and lower count. Believe it or not, a longer period of abstinence is not good either, as older sperm start to degrade and release harmful chemicals that can hurt the good, newer sperm. With long abstinence periods, there will be more nonviable sperm in the sample, which can make the results abnormal. Today, most labs follow the recommended parameters for normal semen analysis given by the World Health Organization (WHO) in 2010.[3] All of the parameters assessed by the semen analysis are important; however, the three parameters that influence a fertility doctor's recommendations the most are concentration (sperm count), motility (how well the sperm move), and morphology (the shape of the sperm). A normal sperm count is 15 million or more sperm per milliliter. A normal motility is 40 percent or more, and a normal morphology is 4 percent or more by Kruger strict morphology. Most men will not have a perfect semen analysis. It is OK to not have a perfect score. Assuming the female testing is normal, slightly abnormal semen parameters can be bypassed by a simple *intrauterine insemination* (IUI) technique. More abnormal parameters will require IVF with *intracytoplasmic sperm injection* (ICSI). I will discuss treatment options in chapter 3. In any case, your doctor can help you determine what mode of treatment is necessary. Men with severe semen parameters will need a full exam and testing by a urologist, so if your semen analysis is severely abnormal, you might be referred to one. A severely abnormal semen analysis can be a sign of a more systemic problem within the body.

3. Reproductive Tract

A normal female reproductive tract is necessary to allow an egg and sperm to meet and fertilize, to transport an embryo to the uterus for implantation, and to incubate an embryo for nine months (see figure 1). Thus, even with normal eggs and sperm, if there are abnormalities within the reproductive tract, achieving pregnancy can be quite difficult. Generally, millions of sperm are deposited in the vagina at the time of intercourse, but only a few hundred will make their way to the egg. After ejaculation into the vagina, the sperm must swim through the *cervix* (the opening to the uterus) and enter the uterus. Only a few hundred sperm will swim past the cervical mucus and enter the uterus. The sperm must then swim from the uterus into the fallopian tube containing the recently ovulated egg. Some of the sperm will lose energy during the swim and not make it to the egg. Timing is critical. The egg emits hormones that attract the sperm to swim toward it, but once ovulated, the egg will survive for only twelve to twenty-four hours. Once the sperm encounter the egg, many sperm will attach to the outer layer of the egg, but only one sperm will pass through this outer layer (the *zona pellucida*) to fertilize the egg.

Fertilization (union of the egg and sperm) occurs in the fallopian tube, and the fertilized egg is called an embryo. The embryo then migrates from the fallopian tube to the uterus. During this migration, the embryo divides (cleaves) and grows. At this point, the fertilized egg is called a *zygote*. The zygote then grows by cell division (cleavage) from one-cell stage to a two-cell stage, a four-cell stage, an eight-cell stage, a *morula* (a solid ball of cells), and a *blastocyst*. The blastocyst is an embryo that has a blastocyst cavity, a *trophoblast* (a layer of cells that will become the placenta), and an *inner cell mass* (comprised of cells that will become the baby). Once in the uterus, the embryo will find a cozy spot to attach to the uterus and begin the implantation process. This is a very complicated process with multiple critical events during which something can go wrong. It is amazing that we can actually reproduce naturally. It is even more amazing that we have figured out how this process works and can manipulate it to help people who are having difficulty conceiving.

There are numerous tests to evaluate the reproductive tract. Three tests frequently done are the *hysterosalpingogram* (HSG), *saline infusion sonogram* (SIS), and *hysteroscopy*. Fertility clinics vary on which they use as the initial test. At one clinic, you might be told that an SIS is fine, but another clinic might require a hysteroscopy before allowing patients to proceed with IVF. I will describe all three tests in detail, but your doctor will recommend which are best for you.

Hysterosalpingogram (HSG): This test utilizes X-rays to visualize the uterus and fallopian tubes. Typically, this test occurs between CD 5 and CD 12 (generally after menstrual bleeding is done but before ovulation) or while on oral contraceptive pills. No sedation is necessary. HSG is a very safe procedure with minimal risks. Most patients do well just by taking 600–800 mg of ibuprofen a couple of hours prior to the procedure. Some clinics may recommend antibiotics prior to the procedure. The HSG is generally done in the office or at a radiology center. The patient will present for the visit, do a urine pregnancy test, sign consent forms, and then undress from the waist down in the procedure room. A speculum exam is performed, similar to a Pap smear. The cervix is prepped with an antiseptic (typically Betadine or Hibiclens), and a small catheter is placed in the cervix. Dye is injected through this catheter into the uterus and, ideally, through the tubes. When the dye goes through the uterus, we can see the shape of the uterus, and when the dye goes through the fallopian tubes, we know that the tubes are open. HSG can suggest abnormal congenital uterine contours such as a *bicornuate uterus*, *septate uterus*, or *unicornuate uterus*. Congenital uterine anomalies are uterine abnormalities that some women are born with and are quite rare; see *Mullerian anomaly* in the glossary for more information. Your doctor will discuss any abnormalities with you. A pelvic magnetic resonance imaging (MRI) or a 3-D saline infusion sonogram can help differentiate among these congenital uterine abnormalities. Sometimes, surgery is necessary to confirm the diagnosis.

Additionally, on the HSG, we can see filling defects in the uterus (areas in the uterus that did not take up the dye), which could be suggestive of *endometrial polyps*, *fibroids*, or *adhesions*. Endometrial polyps and fibroids are generally benign (noncancerous) growths in the uterus that sometimes need to be removed prior to pregnancy. Adhesions (scar tissue) within the uterus can result from prior uterine surgeries and can be seen very well on an HSG. Polyps, fibroids, and adhesions are easily managed surgically.

Normal-appearing fallopian tubes will manifest on the HSG as fine tubal structures that fill with and spill dye. The HSG can also tell us if there is no filling, partial filling, or full filling of the tubes but no spillage. Large, dilated tubes called *hydrosalpinges* can be seen on HSG. These typically result from prior sexually transmitted infections, severe scarring due to endometriosis, or severe scarring due to prior surgeries. They are generally an indication of severe tubal disease. Untreated hydrosalpinges can decrease the chance of pregnancy with IVF by as much as 50 percent.[4] Generally, these tubes are removed or transected surgically prior to embryo transfer with IVF.

Saline infusion sonogram (SIS): Also known as a *hysterosonogram* or *sonohysterogram*, this test utilizes ultrasound as saline is injected into the uterine cavity through a small catheter. An SIS test allows us to visualize the uterus and generally gives us some idea of whether at least one tube is open. Similar to the HSG, this test is typically done between CD 5 and CD 12 as an in-office procedure. The patient presents to the office, signs the consent form, and gives a urine sample for a pregnancy test. She is taken to the ultrasound room and asked to undress from waist down. A speculum exam is performed, similar to a Pap smear; the cervix is cleansed with an antiseptic (typically Betadine or Hibiclens); and a small, thin catheter is placed in the cervix and advanced to the uterus. The speculum is removed, and the transvaginal ultrasound probe is introduced into the vagina. An ultrasound is performed as saline is injected through the catheter. Uterine abnormalities such as fibroids, polyps, or adhesions are easily seen. Congenital Mullerian anomalies (see glossary) can be visualized well using a 3-D ultrasound while injecting the saline. If fluid is seen in the pelvis, it suggests that at least one fallopian tube is open. Very large hydrosalpinges can be seen via an SIS, but smaller-diameter hydrosalpinges are not easily seen.

Hysteroscopy: Hysteroscopy is a procedure in which a small endoscope (called a hysteroscope) is placed in the cervix and gently advanced into the uterus. This can be performed in the office for diagnostic purposes or under anesthesia in a procedure room for diagnosis and treatment. The hysteroscope provides a direct view of the entire uterine cavity and is the gold standard for evaluating the uterus. Hysteroscopies are generally done between CD 5 and CD 12, similar to the HSG and SIS, or while on oral contraceptive pills. These procedures, including those done in the operating room, are generally safe and involve minimal risk. Your doctor will provide informed consent prior to any procedure.

4. Other

Other abnormalities can affect fertility. Fertility doctors will typically perform tests concerning the following.

Thyroid: The thyroid gland regulates many systems in our body. A woman can have low or high thyroid, which are called *hypothyroidism* and *hyperthyroidism* respectively. Hypothyroidism is very common. Women can present with fatigue, hair loss, weight gain, increased sensitivity to cold, changes in the menstrual cycle, constipation, swelling in the neck (growth of the thyroid), or dry skin. Women with hyperthyroidism can present with weight loss, rapid heart rate, increased appetite, nervousness, anxiety, irritability, tremor, sweating, changes in the menstrual cycle, fine and brittle hair, swelling in the neck (growth of the thyroid), fatigue, or increased sensitivity to heat. Thyroid replacement therapy is generally the treatment for hypothyroidism; medications and/or small procedures are generally necessary to treat hyperthyroidism. You will be referred to a medical endocrinologist for management of your thyroid disorder. Occasionally, surgical treatment is necessary.

Prolactin: *Prolactin* is a hormone that typically helps women produce breastmilk after having a baby. However, if prolactin is inappropriately elevated (a condition called *hyperprolactinemia*) in a nonpregnant or nonbreastfeeding woman, it can result in irregular or absent menstrual cycles, *galactorrhea* (milky breast discharge), and, in more severe cases, frequent headaches and loss of peripheral vision. High prolactin levels can result from certain medications or from a small, usually benign tumor in the *pituitary* (a gland in the brain that release hormones). Typically, the treatment for hyperprolactinemia is medication; surgical management is rarely necessary.

Polycystic ovarian syndrome (PCOS): PCOS is a very common endocrine disorder. Based on the 2003 Rotterdam criteria, women with PCOS have been ruled out for other diseases and have two out of three of the following: (1) minimal to no ovulation, (2) clinical or biochemical evidence of hyperandrogenism (e.g., male-pattern hair growth or mildly elevated levels of testosterone), and (3) polycystic ovaries on a sonogram.[5] Women will often present with irregular cycles, lack of ovulation, and, as a result, difficulty conceiving. PCOS is typically associated with an elevation in testosterone, which can manifest as acne or increased hair growth. Some women with PCOS are at an increased risk of type 2 diabetes mellitus (type 2 DM). Thus, an evaluation of blood sugars is warranted in all women with PCOS. Some women with PCOS who are overweight or obese can see a return of normal ovulation after weight loss.

Another much less prevalent but more detrimental disease associated with PCOS is *endometrial hyperplasia*. When women ovulate and get a period every month, the lining of the uterus (the *endometrium*) sheds, and a new lining grows. Women with PCOS do not ovulate regularly and therefore do not shed the endometrial lining regularly. Women with PCOS who are overweight or obese also produce a form of *estrogen* called *estrone* from their fat cells. When the endometrial lining is exposed to constantly mildly elevated levels of estrogen, it is under constant stimulation to grow. It grows excessively thick and can shed unexpectedly, sometimes with large, hemorrhagic bleeds that occasionally require a transfusion due to severe anemia. This very thick endometrial lining can sometimes change its histology and become *hyperplastic*, leading to endometrial hyperplasia. Endometrial hyperplasia is a precursor to endometrial cancer. Endometrial hyperplasia can be detected by a simple *endometrial biopsy* procedure in the office or a *dilation and curettage* (D and C) procedure in the operating room. Early stages of endometrial hyperplasia can be treated medically. Advanced stages may require surgical intervention. Patients with any form of endometrial hyperplasia will need to be seen by a gynecological oncologist.

Women with PCOS are at risk for infertility. This infertility is typically related to the lack of ovulation. Hence, many women first obtain their diagnosis of PCOS when they complain to their doctor of irregular cycles and inability to conceive. If all other infertility testing is normal in a young couple for whom PCOS is the sole source of infertility, simple treatment with medications to induce ovulation will help these patients.

5. Psychological

Too often, the psychological aspect of infertility is overlooked. While stress can lead to difficulties conceiving, it is not usually the only source. Otherwise, a bottle of wine and a beach vacation would cure everyone's fertility problems. Studies have shown that the diagnosis of infertility is as devastating as a diagnosis of cancer.[6] The diagnosis often leads to anxiety and depression. I will devote an entire chapter to the psychological aspect of infertility later in this handbook.

In about 20 percent of couples, the results of the entire testing panel described above come back normal. These couples have *unexplained infertility*. They still have about a 3 percent chance of conceiving naturally per cycle; however,

3 percent is disappointing month after month. Many times, couples with unexplained infertility will need treatment to conceive. Some will conceive easily within the first couple of IUI cycles. Others will need IVF to conceive.

NOTES

1.   G. Lambert-Messerlian et al., "Levels of Antimüllerian Hormone in Serum during the Normal Menstrual Cycle," *Fertility and Sterility* 105, no. 1 (2016): 208–13; A. Overbeek et al., "Intra-Cycle Fluctuations of Anti-Müllerian Hormone in Normal Women with a Regular Cycle: A Re-Analysis," *Reproductive Biomedicine Online* 24, no. 6 (2012): 664–69.

2.   K. Munster, L. Schmidt, and P. Helm, "Length and Variation in the Menstrual Cycle—A Cross-Sectional Study from a Danish County," *British Journal of Obstetrics and Gynaecology* 99, no. 5 (1992): 422–29.

3.   T. G. Cooper et al., "World Health Organization Reference Values for Human Semen Characteristics," *Human Reproduction Update* 16, no. 3 (2010): 231–45.

4.   A. Strandell et al., "Hydrosalpinx and IVF Outcome: A Prospective, Randomized Multicentre Trial in Scandinavia on Salpingectomy Prior to IVF," *Human Reproduction* 14, no. 11 (1999): 2762–69; R. Wainer et al., "Does Hydrosalpinx Reduce the Pregnancy Rate after In Vitro Fertilization?," *Fertility and Sterility* 68, no. 6 (1997): 1022–26; A. S. Blazar et al., "The Impact of Hydrosalpinx on Successful Pregnancy in Tubal Factor Infertility Treated by In Vitro Fertilization," *Fertility and Sterility* 67, no. 3 (1997): 517–20.

5.   Rotterdam ESHRE/ASRM–Sponsored PCOS Consensus Workshop Group, "Revised 2003 Consensus on Diagnostic Criteria and Long-Term Health Risks Related to Polycystic Ovary Syndrome," *Fertility and Sterility* 81, no. 1 (2004): 19–25.

6.   A. D. Domar, P. C. Zuttermeister, and R. Friedman, "The Psychological Impact of Infertility: A Comparison with Patients with Other Medical Conditions," supplement, *Journal of Psychosomatic Obstetrics and Gynaecology* S14 (1993): S45–52.

Three

You Did All the Testing ... What Next?: Your Treatment Options

Typically, your fertility specialist will meet with you once you have completed all the testing. This visit is just as important as the first visit. The physician will review all of your testing and make recommendations based on your testing results. Since we are all different, the treatment recommendations are based on your specific findings and could be different for you when compared to another woman. The following are some examples of treatment options.

1. Natural Conception

Natural conception can be an option for some young couples with good quantity and quality of egg and sperm, predictable ovulatory cycles, and a normal reproductive tract. This typically involves checking ovulation by using ovulation predictor kits (OPKs). Typically, women will start checking ovulation predictor kits around CD 10. There are many good over-the-counter OPKs, but they can vary in price and quality. OPKs involve checking the urine for the ovulation hormone called *luteinizing hormone* (LH). We typically tell patients to check the first urine of the morning for a surge in this hormone. Even though the LH hormone is secreted in pulses, most women have been able to detect a surge with the morning urine sample, as it is the most concentrated. If the hormone is elevated, then that indicates that the woman should ovulate within the next thirty-six hours.[1] During this period, she should have intercourse with her partner. An intrauterine insemination can be done in place of intercourse. Another option for natural conception for women with regular menstrual cycles is to have intercourse every other day from CD 10 to CD 20, with once-per-day intercourse on the two days leading up to ovulation and on the day of ovulation (estimated to be fourteen days prior to the onset of the next menstrual cycle).[2] This ensures that when ovulation happens, there is always sperm available in the woman's reproductive tract to fertilize the egg. This is a good option for women who find the OPKs frustrating or stressful.

2. Intrauterine Insemination (IUI)

An intrauterine insemination has a slightly higher pregnancy success rate than timed intercourse, firstly because IUI will get the sperm closer to the egg, meaning the sperm does not have as far to travel, and secondly because IUI will bypass the cervical mucus. With intercourse, sperm can become trapped in the cervical mucus, which is thick and viscous. A good analogy to sperm swimming in cervical mucus is a fish trying to swim in oil; it is difficult to propel forward in order to get to the destination.

The IUI involves having the male partner give a sperm sample about one to two hours before the IUI. The sperm sample needs to be processed before the insemination. Just like with a semen analysis sample, the male partner should abstain from intercourse for two to five days before giving the sample. The sample is then processed in the lab. For those patients using donor sperm, if they purchased an IUI-ready sample directly from the donor bank, no processing of the sample is necessary. It will merely need to be thawed for insemination. If you purchase a sample from the donor bank that is intracervical insemination (ICI) ready, that sample will also need to be processed before it is used for an intrauterine insemination.

The IUI procedure is similar to a Pap smear. The female partner is asked to undress from the waist down, and a speculum exam is performed. During the speculum exam, a thin catheter is inserted into the cervix and advanced into the uterus. The sample is deposited directly into the uterus via the catheter. Although it is not required, many clinics will have the female partner stay lying down for another ten to fifteen minutes after the IUI. There generally are no restrictions after the IUI; it is also acceptable to go home and have intercourse after an IUI.

3. Monitored Natural Cycles

Some clinics do monitored natural cycles in women with perfect ovulatory menstrual cycles. These women will come in for a baseline sonogram and possibly blood work on CD 2, 3, or 4. If these are normal, they will return around CD 10, 11, or 12 for a repeat sonogram and possibly blood work. If there is a mature follicle, an injection to trigger ovulation is administered. The definition of a mature follicle varies in criteria from clinic to clinic, but most consider a follicle measuring approximately 18–20 mm in diameter to be mature. The "trigger" injection is a version of *human chorionic gonadotropin* (hCG), a hormone found naturally in pregnant women. Very similar to LH in its structure, hCG is capable of triggering the ovulation process like LH. hCG drugs commonly used today include Ovidrel, Novarel, and Pregnyl. Once the trigger is administered, the female patient can have timed intercourse or do an IUI about twenty-four to thirty-six hours later. If the trigger is not given, a woman will ovulate spontaneously. Spontaneous ovulation is less predictable than utilizing hCG triggers and can make the timing of intercourse or IUI less accurate. Sometimes, when a patient returns for the sonogram and blood work on CD 10–12, there is a follicle that is growing but not yet mature. The woman will be asked to return in a few days for a repeat sonogram in order to give the follicle a few more days to grow and achieve maturity.

4. Ovulation Induction with Oral Medications

Oral medications commonly used for ovulation induction include clomiphene citrate (Clomid) and letrozole (Femara). These medications are typically taken for five days. Some clinics will have the patient take the pills on CDs 3–7, CDs 4–8, or CDs 5–9. Studies have shown no significant differences regarding ovulation and pregnancy rates with regard to which five days the meds are taken.[3] Generally, the earlier in the cycle a woman takes the medications and/or the higher the dose, the greater her chances of recruiting more follicles (possible eggs) that may ovulate. The goal is to have one to two follicles ovulate in order to conceive. Too many follicles ovulating at the same time can increase the chances of multiples. In many fertility practices, ovulation induction cycles are monitored with sonograms a few times during the cycle. Generally, a woman will come in for a baseline sonogram and possibly blood work on CD 2, 3, or 4. If these results are normal, she will take the five days of oral medications. Commonly, she will return for a sonogram on CD 10, 11, or 12. If there is a mature follicle, the hCG trigger shot will be given, and either timed intercourse or IUI can be done. If the follicle is growing but not mature at the time of the sonogram on CD 10, 11, or 12, then the woman will return for a repeat sonogram in a few days in order to give the follicle a few more days to mature.

Women with PCOS can have *anovulation* (lack of ovulation) or *oligoovulation* (infrequent ovulation). In a young couple where PCOS-related anovulation is the only source of infertility, ovulation induction with oral medications is typically a first-line treatment. Approximately 60–85 percent of women with PCOS will ovulate in response to taking clomiphene citrate; however, the other 15–40 percent will fail to ovulate after receiving a high dose of 150 mg daily of clomiphene citrate. This is sometimes called *clomiphene-resistant PCOS*.[4] This remaining 15–40 percent should consider moving on to ovulation induction with gonadotropin injections or directly to IVF.

5. Ovulation Induction with Gonadotropin Injections

Injectable medications currently used for ovulation induction in the United States include Follistim, Gonal F, and Menopur. There are many more injectable medications used throughout the world under various brand names, but there is not much difference in the medications in terms of their efficacy. The injectable medications are either purified or recombinant (engineered in the lab) versions of two hormones: follicle stimulating hormone (FSH) and luteinizing hormone (LH). Both of these hormones are naturally produced by our pituitary gland, which stimulates a woman's ovaries to produce mature follicles containing eggs; the follicles in turn make the hormones estradiol (a form of estrogen) and progesterone. Therefore, these injectable hormones will stimulate ovaries to produce eggs. In the past, the injections were taken intramuscularly, but now they can be taken subcutaneously (just under the skin). Subcutaneous administration uses shorter, thinner needles, and the needle does not have to go in as deep, so there is less pain. You will become an expert at giving yourself shots after undergoing infertility treatments.

Even though IVF is often in the news and gets a bad reputation for pregnancies with higher-order multiples (triplets or higher), ovulation induction with injections causes the highest rate of multiples. With IVF, doctors can control the number of embryos they return to the uterus (and therefore the chance of multiples). Injectable ovulation induction medications will stimulate the ovaries to make eggs and ovulate them. Women who overstimulate and recruit three or more follicles are at the highest risk for a higher-order multiple pregnancy.

Most women will utilize the injectables for approximately ten days. This can be a very busy ten days for these women. In addition to taking these medications daily, women will come to the doctor's office every two to three days for monitoring, which consists of ultrasounds to evaluate follicle growth and maturation as well as blood testing to evaluate various hormones. Once the follicles (eggs) are ready, the woman will take the hCG trigger shot and either do timed intercourse or an IUI. If her doctor sees that she is making too many eggs that cycle, the doctor may cancel the cycle. While a cancelled cycle can be a disappointment, high-order multiples are unsafe pregnancies that can result in preterm labor, bed rest for many months, preterm deliveries, and, potentially, long-term disabilities in the children due to preterm births.

6. In Vitro Fertilization (IVF)

All the forms of conception mentioned thus far refer to conception happening within the female reproductive tract. On the other hand, IVF involves conception happening outside the female reproductive tract. The eggs and sperm are united in the lab to form the embryo. In some cases, birth control pills are taken for a few weeks before beginning the IVF stimulation process. The birth control pills suppress the ovaries, organize the follicles, and are used to start the injectable medications in a timely manner. The injections used for IVF are very similar to those used for the ovulation induction with gonadotropin injection cycles, but at higher dosages. With ovulation induction cycles, the goal is to get one to two follicles to mature, whereas with IVF, the goal is to recruit ten to fifteen follicles in a cycle. The woman will take the injections for approximately nine to twelve days.

QUESTION:

Will IVF decrease the number of eggs I have in my lifetime and put me in early menopause?

ANSWER:

IVF does not deplete your lifetime eggs or put you in early menopause. IVF takes advantage of the same amount of eggs that your body would have produced that cycle. In a natural cycle, the woman will start off with a few follicles (each follicle contains an egg) at the beginning of the cycle. All but one of these follicles will regress and are permanently gone. This one remaining follicle will grow and mature, becoming the *dominant follicle* and releasing (ovulating) the egg that cycle. The goal of the injectable medications with IVF is to promote all the follicles at the start of the cycle to grow and mature.

QUESTION:
What happens at the IVF egg retrieval?

ANSWER:
Before a woman can ovulate spontaneously in an IVF cycle, the eggs are retrieved. The egg retrieval is an outpatient, same-day surgical procedure. Approximately thirty-four to thirty-eight hours prior to the retrieval, the woman will take a trigger shot. Typical trigger shots are leuprolide acetate and hCG. Use of leuprolide acetate is becoming more common, as it reduces the risk of complications from *ovarian hyper-stimulation syndrome* (OHSS). OHSS is a medical condition that usually happens after retrieval or after a *fresh embryo transfer* in which pregnancy is achieved. (See the glossary for more information.) When a woman produces too many eggs, her estrogen levels rise, which causes a release of other hormones within the body. The release of these other hormones can cause fluid to collect in the pelvis and/or lungs and increases the risk of blood clots and electrolyte (salt) abnormalities in the blood. Fluid in the pelvis can cause

pain and pressure and may need to be removed. Fluid in the lungs can cause difficulty breathing and may also need to be removed. Electrolyte abnormalities in the blood may need to be corrected with intravenous fluids. Rarely, blood clots can develop in the legs and/or lungs, which can be life threatening. OHSS is a self-limiting disease, which means it always resolves with time, so we manage the symptoms of OHSS while the body heals itself. As long as there is no embryo transfer, the symptoms of OHSS significantly improve with the start of the next menses following the egg retrieval.

Prior to the egg retrieval, the woman should not eat or drink anything after midnight the night before the procedure; eight hours of fasting is needed, similar to many other procedures in which anesthesia will be administered. Typically, she will arrive one hour prior to her procedure time for preparation, which generally includes getting intravenous fluids started and discussing her care with the nursing staff, anesthesiologist, and fertility specialist. In the procedure room, the anesthesiologist will give her medications to put her to sleep. This is a deep sleep, so the woman will not feel pain or have any memory of the procedure, but she will typically breathe on her own. You can discuss with the anesthesiologist which medications they will use for you. Some centers require that certain patients with medical conditions meet with an anesthesiologist before starting the IVF process to make sure they are good candidates for anesthesia. If you are not a good anesthesia candidate, then you should not do IVF. Most patients, however, are healthy young women who just want to have a baby; therefore, the IVF process is of minimal burden to their bodies.

After anesthesia has been administered, the woman is prepped for the procedure. Her legs are placed in stirrups, and her pelvic area is cleansed before starting the procedure. The procedure is officially named a *transvaginal oocyte retrieval* (TVOR). The reason for the name TVOR is that the eggs are removed vaginally, with no incisions on the abdomen. A transvaginal ultrasound is placed in the vagina and used to visualize the follicles. (Remember: in theory, each follicle contains an egg.) A needle is attached to the ultrasound probe. We use the ultrasound to show us where to put the needle. The needle, which is connected to a suction tube, will traverse the vaginal wall and enter directly into the ovary. The fluid in the follicle is aspirated into the needle and suction tube and then collected into a test tube, which is handed to the embryologist. The embryologist will typically pour the fluid from the test tube into a petri dish (a small laboratory bowl) and, under the microscope, search for eggs in the fluid. The eggs are then removed from the fluid and placed in a separate petri dish. Once the procedure is complete, the woman is awakened and taken to the recovery room. Generally, TVOR procedures are safe, with a less than 1 percent risk of bleeding, infection, excessive pain, or anesthesia complications.

QUESTION:

How many eggs will I obtain at the egg retrieval?

ANSWER:

Most but not all follicles will produce an egg at the time of retrieval. Clinics and physicians may differ in their trigger criteria, which can also vary from patient to patient depending on ovarian reserve. Follicles under 12 mm at the time of trigger will rarely produce a mature egg. Similarly, very large follicles may not release an egg. A good predictor of the number of eggs anticipated at the retrieval is the number of 15–22 mm follicles that you have on the day of the trigger shot. Generally, younger women make more eggs than women of a more advanced reproductive age. We are all different, so there are some very young women with few eggs and women of advanced reproductive age with many eggs who do not fit the typical pattern of declining egg quantity with age.

QUESTION:

What happens after the retrieval?

ANSWER:

At the timing of writing this book, the field of reproductive endocrinology and infertility (REI) is moving toward *frozen embryo transfer* (FET) (see glossary). With typical FET cycles, the transfer is delayed after the retrieval. Once the eggs are retrieved, they are fertilized with sperm. The eggs can be fertilized with standard insemination or with intracytoplasmic sperm injection (ICSI). Standard insemination involves putting the eggs and sperm together in a petri dish and allowing the sperm to naturally fertilize the eggs. ICSI involves directly injecting a single sperm into a single egg. Standard insemination is typically done with sperm from a sample with normal semen parameters. Essentially, ICSI is done for all other forms of fertilization, including with sperm from an abnormal sample; with sperm retrieved directly from the testicles; in some cases, in which *preimplantation genetic testing* (PGT) will be done (see glossary); and in some cases of frozen semen samples. Once the eggs are fertilized, they are incubated overnight and checked the next day. Fertilization (which eggs took up the sperm correctly) is evaluated the next day. The fertilized eggs are now called zygotes, which will typically grow out until the blastocyst stage (five to seven days after the egg retrieval). The embryos are frozen or cryopreserved at the blastocyst stage and can later be used for a frozen embryo transfer (FET). Some patients may request preimplantation genetic testing (PGT), which involves biopsying the blastocyst before freezing. Very few clinics today will freeze embryos at the zygote stage (one day after retrieval) or the six- to eight-cell stage (three days post retrieval). Because FETs utilizing blastocysts are more commonly done today, the woman is done for a few weeks after the egg retrieval and will wait for her next menses. The next menses typically will start within two weeks of the retrieval, after which the FET cycle can be planned.

QUESTION:

What is preimplantation genetic testing?

ANSWER:

Preimplantation genetic testing (PGT) involves a genetic evaluation of the embryos. There are various forms of PGT, but PGT-A (aneuploidy screening) is the most common form. All forms of PGT involve taking approximately five cells from the *trophectoderm* (the part of the blastocyst that will become the placenta). The actual inner cell mass (the part of the blastocyst that will become the baby) is not biopsied. In theory, the trophectoderm and the inner cell mass have the same genetic makeup; therefore, the genetic results of the trophectoderm should be indicative of the genetic makeup of the inner cell mass. PGT-A involves evaluating the embryo for *aneuploidy*. Generally, all of our cells have forty-six *chromosomes* (twenty-three pairs). In females, the chromosomal content of the cells is 46XX, and in males, it's 46XY. Aneuploidy is the presence of an abnormal number of chromosomes or gene regions in a cell. Embryos made up of *aneuploid* cells will typically not implant or will result in miscarriage. The most common condition in which an aneuploid embryo makes it to delivery is Down syndrome (trisomy 21), in which the embryo has forty-seven chromosomes, with three copies of chromosome 21 instead of two. PGT-M (monogenic) involves testing for single-gene disorders. For example, cystic fibrosis is a very common single-gene disorder in our population. It is an autosomal recessive trait, meaning that the offspring must inherit an abnormal copy from the father and also an abnormal copy from the mother. When a parent carries an abnormal gene and wants to prevent passing this gene down to the next generation, PGT-M is utilized. Embryos that do not carry the abnormal gene are preferred for transfer to the uterus.

7. Frozen Embryo Transfer (FET)

Frozen embryo transfer (FET) involves thawing the embryo and transferring it to the uterus. An FET cycle generally involves the female taking two to three weeks of estrogen to prepare the lining of the uterus. This estrogen comes in various forms, including oral, vaginal, transdermal, and intramuscular, although the drugs used can vary based on the patient and the clinic. The woman will come in to the office about once per week to make sure that the uterine lining (*endometrium*) is growing in response to the estrogen. Once the uterine lining is thick enough, progesterone is started. Progesterone is needed to mimic what would happen in a natural cycle after ovulation and before implantation. Progesterone supplementation is typically continued until the end of the first trimester.

After a few days of progesterone, the woman will come back to the clinic for the embryo transfer. The embryo is typically thawed a few hours prior to the procedure. The woman is typically allowed to eat and drink prior to the transfer, since generally no anesthesia is given, and is asked to come to the clinic with a full bladder. This is necessary because an abdominal ultrasound will be done during the transfer process. The full bladder allows us to see the uterus well on the sonogram and helps to straighten out the angle between the uterus and cervix, making navigation with the transfer catheter easier. When she arrives, the patient will speak to the embryologist, who will confirm the patient and the embryo. If PGT was performed, those results are available for discussion. The woman is then taken back to the procedure room and undresses from the waist down. A speculum is placed in the vagina, and the cervix is cleansed. An introductory catheter is then placed at the cervix and advanced into the uterus. We use the ultrasound to tell us how far to go with the catheter. A second catheter containing the embryo is inserted through the introductory catheter to place the embryo into the uterus. Both catheters are then removed, and the embryologist will flush the inner catheter under the microscope to make sure that the embryo did not stick to that catheter. Once the embryologist confirms that the catheter is clear, the speculum is removed from the vagina. Recent publications support no bedrest immediately after the transfer, but many clinics may have the woman stay lying down for approximately thirty minutes before leaving the clinic.[5] Some will also recommend that the woman not do any heavy exertion, such as high aerobic activity or lifting anything greater than ten pounds, for a couple of days following the transfer. The pregnancy test will be performed about nine to twelve days following the FET.

8. Fresh Embryo Transfer

A *fresh embryo transfer* typically involves returning the embryo or embryos to the uterus just a few days after the retrieval without freezing them. Fresh embryo transfers are not done frequently today. Many clinics that do predominantly FET will only do fresh embryo transfers for patients who have embryos of low quantity and quality. Essentially, these are embryos that, if we waited until the blastocyst stage, would all stop growing, meaning there would therefore be no embryos for transfer.

KNOWING YOUR OPTIONS

QUESTION:

My doctor gave me several options for fertility treatments, as listed above. How do I know which one is right for me?

ANSWER:

Your doctor will make recommendations for treatment based on your testing. For example, if your thyroid is abnormal, your doctor will recommend that your thyroid be treated first before starting fertility treatment. Some patients might even get pregnant naturally if that was their only problem. If you have abnormal fallopian tubes or severely abnormal sperm, your doctor will recommend IVF since the other forms of treatment will be less helpful. If you have unexplained infertility, you can try any of the forms of treatments listed above;

however, the success rates differ for each form of treatment in a couple with unexplained infertility.

No Treatment	1.3–4.1%
IUI	3.8%
Clomiphene Citrate	5.6%
Clomiphene Citrate with IUI	8.3%
Gonadotropins	7.7%
Gonadotropins with IUI	17.1%
IVF	20.7% (1998) Can be as high as more than 70% depending on prognosis of the couple, IVF lab, etc. (2016)

Table 1: Treatment success rates for patients with unexplained infertility.[6]

In the past, we measured the effectiveness of treatment by pregnancy success rate, but since some pregnancies can result in miscarriages, we now measure by live birth rate. This makes sense since the goal of the patient is to have a baby to take home. In 1998, the pregnancy success rate for IVF was published as 20.7 percent.[7] Since then, IVF technology has improved. Now, the rate of live births in young healthy patients with IVF is as high as 70 percent or more.[8] This varies by lab and other prognostic criteria specific to each couple.

Because of the excellent IVF pregnancy success rate that we have today, many patients electively choose to forgo simpler forms of treatment and pursue IVF as the initial form of treatment.

QUESTION:

How do my finances affect which fertility treatment I choose?

ANSWER:

Most insurance plans will cover the diagnostic testing for infertility, but only a small percentage of insurance plans cover treatment. It is difficult enough to want a child and not be able to conceive, but adding a financial burden can make the process even more overwhelming. Once you have met the doctor and discussed treatment options, you should meet the financial counselor to discuss cost, which can influence the treatment option you choose. Some insurance plans may require that you do several IUI cycles before they pay for an IVF cycle. If you have a qualifier for IVF (such as both tubes being blocked or severe male factor), then the insurance plan may allow you to move directly to IVF. Some insurance plans have a lifetime maximum of fertility treatment coverage, so it may be beneficial to go directly to IVF in these scenarios rather than waste your treatment coverage on less successful forms of treatment. Most insurance plans will not pay for IVF if either partner has had any form of voluntary sterilization, such as a tubal ligation or vasectomy. Keep in mind that insurance coverage varies based on your plan and also by state. Some states are called mandated states, meaning they are required by law to provide some type of insurance coverage for fertility. Knowing your financial options is just as important as knowing your medical options.

NOTES

1. M. A. Fritz and L. Speroff, *Clinical Gynecologic Endocrinology and Infertility* (Philadelphia: Lippincott Williams & Wilkins, 2011), 228.

2. Practice Committee of the American Society for Reproductive Medicine, "Optimizing Natural Fertility," supplement, *Fertility and Sterility* 90, no. S5 (2008): S1–S6.

3. N. Ghomian, A. Khosravi, and N. Mousavifar, "A Randomized Clinical Trial on Comparing the Cycle Characteristics of Two Different Initiation Days of Letrozole Treatment in Clomiphene Citrate Resistant PCOS Patients in IUI Cycles," *International Journal of Fertility and Sterility* 9, no. 1 (2015): 17–26.

4. H. A. Hashim, T. Shokeir, and A. Badawy, "Letrozole Versus Combined Metformin and Clomiphene Citrate for Ovulation Induction in Clomiphene-Resistant Women with Polycystic Ovary Syndrome: A Randomized Control Trial," *Fertility and Sterility* 94, no. 4 (2010): 1405–09.

5. K. J. Purcell et al., "Bed Rest after Embryo Transfer: A Randomized Controlled Trial," *Fertility and Sterility* 87, no. 6 (2007): 1322–26.

6. D. S. Guzick et al., "Efficacy of Treatment for Unexplained Infertility," *Fertility and Sterility* 70, no. 2 (1998): 207–13; "Best IVF Clinics in United States for Women Under 35 Using Thawed Embryos," Fertility Success Rates, TD Media, https://fertilitysuccessrates.com/report/United-States/women-under-35/thawed/data.html.

7. Guzick, "Efficacy of Treatment for Unexplained Infertility."

8. "Best IVF Clinics in United States."

Four

Third-Party Reproduction

QUESTION:
What is third-party reproduction?

ANSWER:
Sometimes, your testing results can show that one of the three big components (eggs, sperm, and reproductive tract) has very poor function. Some couples might be missing a component (e.g., same-sex couples, single parents, or someone with an absent or severely abnormal uterus), so to have a baby, they will need eggs, sperm, and/or a reproductive tract from someone else. This is difficult news to receive, but there are options available if you choose to utilize them. Let us review each in detail.

1. Donor Egg
Using a donor egg means that you will need to utilize eggs from another woman. The donor is typically a woman in her twenties or early thirties whose ovarian-reserve testing is outstanding. Most female patients in the United States will choose

an *anonymous donor*. Occasionally, a female patient will ask a sister or friend to donate eggs; this is called a *known donor*. Known donors can be older, with acceptable ovarian reserve, when compared to the strict requirements for anonymous donors. However, known donors are well known to the couple because they chose this donor for a particular reason, such as a relative with a similar genetic makeup or a friend with known physical and personality characteristics. A couple is always counseled regarding the advantages and disadvantages of using a known donor. All parties are required to undergo psychological screening to assess whether they are comfortable with the egg donation process. Use of anonymous donors provides an emotional separation that isn't possible when using a friend or relative. The majority of patients typically like that separation, but if known donation is right for you, that is available. In donor IVF cycles, all parties will work with an attorney to delineate parental rights before the medical process can begin.

Choosing a donor egg as a means of having a child can be difficult for some couples. After all, you are choosing one half of your child's *DNA* (deoxyribonucleic acid). Many female patients will choose a donor that is of the same ethnic origin with similar physical features. Donors typically write short paragraphs in their profiles regarding why they wanted to be donors. These essays can give you insight into the donor's personality and can be very beneficial. Several patients have told me that these short paragraphs allow them to have an emotional connection to someone who was kind enough to donate eggs—someone they will never meet. Some patients will choose a donor who has donated in the past and has proven success. This is not necessary since anonymous donors are so well tested and have good ovarian reserve. Additionally, a donor's success in the past does not guarantee you a pregnancy.

The donor will take the gonadotropin injections for approximately ten days, after which she will undergo the egg retrieval. Once the eggs are retrieved, they are fertilized with sperm from the male partner. Clinics will set the schedule so that the male partner and the donor never encounter each other. Many clinics will have the male partner freeze sperm ahead of time to simplify the process. The embryos are typically grown out until the blastocyst stage. In the past, the donor's IVF cycle was synchronized with the recipient's uterine preparation cycle. Essentially, the hormonal environment of the donor was complementary to that of the recipient. Once the blastocysts were ready, they were transferred to the recipient's uterus. Now that FET cycles are successful, predominantly due to *vitrification* (a fast method of freezing embryos), the recipient can wait a few weeks or months before doing the transfer. This allows for PGT testing and makes scheduling more convenient for both donor and recipient. For example, the donor can do the IVF cycle in the summer before going back to school in the fall, and the recipient can have one last fantastic summer vacation before getting pregnant.

Donor egg banks are now becoming more popular and successful. Instead of choosing a donor, who then undergoes an IVF cycle after being chosen, you choose eggs from a donor who has already been screened and whose eggs have already been retrieved and frozen. Essentially, you purchase the eggs directly from the egg bank, and the eggs are shipped frozen to the fertility clinic of your choice. There are two possible paths for the transfer. Option one: you start to prepare the lining of your uterus; the eggs are thawed and fertilized with sperm; the embryos are grown out to the blastocyst stage; and then they are transferred. Option two: the eggs are thawed and fertilized with sperm; the embryos are grown to the blastocyst stage. If PGT-A testing is desired, the biopsy can be done prior to freezing the embryos. Once the PGT-A results have been received, the recipient starts a cycle to prepare the uterus; and then the desirable embryo(s) are transferred.

A frozen donor egg cycle is less expensive than a fresh donor egg cycle. With a fresh donor egg cycle, one recipient pays for that donor screening and IVF cycle, but then all the eggs and resulting embryos belong to that recipient. With frozen donor eggs, the donors have already been prescreened, the retrieval has been completed, and the eggs have been frozen. The eggs from one donor cycle are then split into batches of approximately six to nine eggs per batch and sold to several recipients. It is estimated that one "batch" of eggs will yield one to two blastocysts for transfer. Hence, the screening and IVF-cycle costs for that donor are split among several recipients, which makes a frozen donor egg cycle less expensive per recipient. Because a smaller batch of eggs is distributed to each recipient with a frozen donor egg cycle than with a fresh donor egg cycle, there is typically little to no surplus of frozen embryos. For couples with religious concerns about a surplus of frozen embryos, doing a frozen donor egg cycle is more advantageous. For couples who want to have more than one pregnancy with biologically related siblings, having a surplus of frozen embryos for subsequent pregnancies is more advantageous. Studies have shown that frozen donor eggs have pregnancy rates equivalent to fresh donor eggs.[1] Thus, cost and the need to have a surplus of frozen embryos are typically the determining factors when a couple is deciding whether to do a fresh donor egg cycle or a frozen one. In the near future, it is likely that frozen donor egg cycles will be more frequently utilized than fresh ones due to the convenience and ease of utilization.

2. Donor Sperm

We have been utilizing donor sperm for decades. While a donor egg cycle is a very intricate, complex process, sperm donation is relatively simple. There are many reputable banks in the country from which donor sperm can be purchased. Generally, when a male decides that he wants to be a donor, he fills out a long questionnaire. Some males are found to be ineligible based on their answers. The ones who are eligible are then screened for multiple infectious diseases, undergo psychological screening, and also give a semen sample. The semen sample is placed in a quarantine bank for six months. The donor returns in six months to repeat the infectious disease testing. If the repeat infectious disease testing is normal, then the quarantined sample can be released for the public to purchase.

Cytomegalovirus (CMV) is a very common virus that causes "flu-like" symptoms. More than half of the world's population has been exposed to CMV by coming in contact with bodily fluids (such as saliva, tears, blood, semen, urine, mucus, breast milk, or vaginal fluids) from someone who has an active infection. Generally, once a person has had CMV, that person has lifelong immunity. If a nonimmune pregnant woman contracts the virus, there is a risk of transmission to the baby, which can possibly result in birth defects, hearing loss, neurological abnormalities, or loss of the pregnancy. Donor sperm banks test the donors for CMV, as there is a theoretical risk that a semen sample from a CMV-positive donor could cause a nonimmune recipient to contract CMV, thus increasing the risks to the pregnancy. Some fertility clinics will test the female patient to see if she is immune to CMV. If she is immune to CMV, she can use sperm from a donor who is positive or negative for CMV. If the woman is not immune to CMV, she should use CMV-negative sperm.

Traditionally, sperm donations have been anonymous. The websites of donor sperm *cryobanks* (where sperm cells are frozen and stored) allow you to create searches for your donor sperm; you can create multiple wish lists to help you find your favorite donor. Search criteria include height, hair color, eye color, ethnicity, educational level, ancestry, religion, and many other parameters. It can take days—sometimes weeks—to find the right donor. Once the right donor has been selected, the sperm sample is shipped frozen to the fertility clinic of your choice. As mentioned earlier, you want to buy an IUI-ready sample if you intend to do an IUI procedure. These samples generally come with a quantity guarantee. If you intend to do an IUI procedure and purchase an ICI-ready sample, the ICI sample will be washed by the fertility clinic. For IVF, an IUI-ready, ICI-ready, or IVF-ready sample can be used since the sample generally undergoes additional preparation before fertilization of the egg with ICSI. In addition to *anonymous donations*, many sperm banks provide a certain percentage of their samples as *open donations*. These specific sperm donors are open to having a resulting offspring contact them once that offspring reaches age eighteen or older.

3. Gestational Carriers

Some women who were born without a uterus, have had a hysterectomy, or have a serious medical condition cannot carry a pregnancy. These women will do IVF to create the embryo and then have the embryo transferred to a *gestational carrier*. Gestational carriers are also an option for males in a same-sex couple who want to be parents. The term *traditional surrogacy* refers to a situation in which the egg is from the same person as the uterus that is being used to carry the pregnancy. Colloquially, the term *surrogate* often means *gestational surrogate or gestational carrier*, meaning the recipient is not biologically related to the embryo. In the United States today, gestational surrogacy is more commonly used, whereas traditional surrogacy is rarely used because it is a more challenging scenario legally and ethically. Certain countries, and even certain states within the United States, legally prohibit the use of gestational carriers. Gestational carriers are typically women of good health who have carried their own children and are done having more children of their own but want to be pregnant to help others become parents.

The decision to use a surrogate can be very difficult for a woman, since many women feel inadequate if they cannot carry their own child. Once a woman is emotionally ready to conceive via a gestational carrier, she must find one. Some women are fortunate enough to have a family member or friend who is willing to carry their child. However, most women will either select a surrogate from an agency or meet a surrogate through one of the many websites and online chats where surrogates and intended parents connect. The advantage of using an agency is that the gestational carrier has been interviewed and vetted to some degree by a third party (i.e., the agency). However, the major disadvantage of using an agency is that agency fees are very expensive. These agency fees are direct payments to the agency that do not count toward the surrogacy cycle. Once a surrogate has been selected, she will go to the fertility clinic for an evaluation. If the surrogate's evaluation demonstrates that she is medically fit to be a gestational carrier, then it is time to get psychological evaluations and sign legal agreements. All parties should undergo the psychological evaluation, including the surrogate's partner, to be sure that they are comfortable with their partner carrying a pregnancy for another couple. The surrogate's partner is part of her support system and should be available to help her during the pregnancy. Therefore, it is important that they are on board with this process. The legal documents clearly delineate who the legal parents are, establish guidelines for potential events during pregnancy, and outline a payment schedule for the surrogate.

Once medical clearance, psychological evaluation, and legal documents have been completed, it is time to start the medical process. Because many clinics have moved to FET cycles and many intended parents will do PGT testing, transfer to the surrogate is a standard FET cycle. All parties then wait for the pregnancy test, typically performed about a week and half after the transfer. The surrogate undergoes blood testing for the pregnancy hormone. Once the pregnancy hormone is high enough, there will be a sonogram to confirm the pregnancy, then subsequent prenatal care with an obstetrician. In the past and in some states currently, the birth certificate was in the name of the surrogate and the intended parents had to adopt their child. Now, in other states, the intended parents can obtain a prebirth order during the second trimester and present this prebirth order to hospital officials at the time of delivery to have their names printed on the birth certificate.

4. Reciprocal IVF

Reciprocal IVF is a term typically used when a female same-sex couple wants to have a child together using the eggs of one female, which are fertilized with donor sperm and then transferred to the other female partner. This is a fantastic way to have both partners involved in making a baby. Reciprocal IVF is also a good option when one partner cannot or does not want to carry the pregnancy. For example, I have worked with several female same-sex couples who have transferred good *euploid* embryos (embryos with the right number of chromosomes or gene regions) that nonetheless resulted in recurrent negative pregnancy tests or recurrent miscarriages. Those that agreed to then have the other partner try to carry the pregnancy have been successful. Thus, having another uterus as an option can be beneficial.

5. Uterine Transplant

Uterine transplant clinical trials are presently being studied in the United States for women who were born without a uterus but are otherwise healthy enough to carry their own child. It is a costly, detailed process involving surgical procedures and immunosuppressive drugs, but for some women, carrying their own child is an emotional journey. Typically, since these women have ovaries but do not have a uterus, embryos are made and frozen via the IVF process. The woman is placed on a transplant list and eventually matched to a donor. In addition to receiving a uterine transplant, the woman is placed on immunosuppressive therapy to make sure that her body does not reject the uterus. Once it has been determined that her body did not reject the uterus, the embryo transfer (generally FET) will take place. The fetus will grow until term and, commonly, will be delivered by cesarean section. There have been several live births worldwide following uterine transplants, with the first in the United States announced in December 2017 at Baylor University Medical Center in Dallas, Texas.[2] Here in the United States, uterine transplantation is only available under clinical trials and therefore is not ready for routine use.

6. Adoption

Adoption is another option. There are thousands of children in the United States—and many more in countries throughout the world—who need a loving family to take care of them. A couple needs to be comfortable with adoption before pursuing this option. If having a biological child is essential, then adoption will not be successful. However, many intended parents truly feel that being a parent comes from the nurturing and love that a parent can provide, not from just the ability to conceive a child. Adoption is right for these intended parents. Couples will typically go through a certified agency to adopt an infant or child. Certified agencies will often do a background check on you and a home study visit to see whether you will be able to provide a healthy, nurturing environment to an infant or child. The agency can help you decide whether you want to do a domestic adoption, international adoption, or foster adoption. There are adoption fees due to the amount of support and counseling offered both to adoptive families and to birth parents. In some cases, open adoption is an option, allowing some form of contact between the child and the birth parents. Ways in which a child can benefit from an open adoption include the opportunity to build a relationship with the birth parents, access to the medical and genetic history of the birth parents, and security in one's own identity, since the child knows how they came to be.

NOTES

1. J. A. Grifo and N. Noyes, "Delivery Rate Using Cryopreserved Oocytes Is Comparable to Conventional In Vitro Fertilization Using Fresh Oocytes: Potential Fertility Preservation for Female Cancer Patients," *Fertility and Sterility* 93, no. 2 (2010): 391–96; K. M. Trokoudes, C. Pavlides, and X. Zhang, "Comparison Outcome of Fresh and Vitrified Donor Oocytes in an Egg-Sharing Donation Program," *Fertility and Sterility* 95, no. 6 (1996): 1996–2000.

2. Alexandra Sifferlin, "Exclusive: First U.S. Baby Born after a Uterus Transplant," *Time*, December 1, 2017, http://time.com/5044565/ exclusive-first-u-s-baby-born-after-a-uterus-transplant.

Five

Fertility Preservation

Fertility preservation is an option for anyone who wants to conceive in the future but is not ready to be a parent soon. Today, both oocytes (eggs) and sperm are routinely frozen via a method called vitrification. Vitrification is a way of rapidly freezing the eggs and sperm. It has a better thaw rate for specimens when compared to slow freezing, which is less commonly done today. *Sperm cryopreservation* involves the male producing the sample into a cup. The sample is then processed, and the sperm is frozen. *Oocyte cryopreservation* is not as simple, as it requires the woman to do the steps of IVF up to egg retrieval. After the egg retrieval, the eggs are not fertilized. Instead, they are cryopreserved (frozen). For both eggs and sperm, the better the quantity and quality of the sample before freezing, the better the thaw rate, which is extremely important for women freezing eggs. The younger a woman is at the time of freezing, the higher her chances of freezing a large number of good-quality eggs. Frozen eggs have similar pregnancy rates when compared to fresh eggs in healthy young women.[1] Unfortunately, many women presently do not consider oocyte cryopreservation until they are older. Awareness has improved, with some people holding "egg freezing parties" and some employers offering fertility preservation to employees in their benefits packages. Oocyte and sperm cryopreservation can be done for anyone who electively wants to delay childbearing or who is about to start medications potentially toxic to oocytes or sperm, such as chemotherapy.

NOTES

1. J. A. Grifo and N. Noyes, "Delivery Rate Using Cryopreserved Oocytes Is Comparable to Conventional In Vitro Fertilization Using Fresh Oocytes: Potential Fertility Preservation for Female Cancer Patients," *Fertility and Sterility* 93, no. 2 (2010): 391–96; K. M. Trokoudes, C. Pavlides, and X. Zhang, "Comparison Outcome of Fresh and Vitrified Donor Oocytes in an Egg-Sharing Donation Program," *Fertility and Sterility* 95, no. 6 (1996): 1996–2000.

Six

Recurrent Pregnancy Loss

The American Society for Reproductive Medicine (ASRM) has defined *recurrent pregnancy loss* (RPL) as two or more failed clinical pregnancies.[1] A clinical pregnancy is one that is identified on a sonogram or on a pathology report after the pregnancy is lost. Physicians typically do an RPL evaluation after two or more losses. Additionally, some physicians will do the evaluation testing in patients who have lost pregnancies after ten weeks of gestation. This is because pregnancy losses after ten weeks are not common. Typically, patients who've had one miscarriage do not need to undergo RPL testing because incidental miscarriages are relatively common. Therefore, an RPL evaluation will likely not be helpful after a single miscarriage at fewer than ten weeks of gestation.

A chromosomally abnormal embryo, called an aneuploid embryo, is the most commonly known cause of RPL. Almost all aneuploid embryos result from mistakes in cell division that occur within the first weeks after conception. Humans are very inefficient at reproduction; it is estimated that 34.5 percent of embryos are aneuploidy in women at age thirty-five and 58.2 percent at age forty. This percentage continues to increase with age.[2] Most of these aneuploid embryos will never implant, but the ones that do are usually lost in miscarriage. Abnormalities in the parents' chromosomes are the source of about 2–8 percent of RPL.[3] Most of these parental chromosomal abnormalities are *balanced translocations*, which means that all the chromosomes are present but a section of one chromosome is attached to another chromosome. When the egg or sperm of the parent who has a balanced translocation is used to create an embryo, the genetic material can become unbalanced and prone to a miscarriage.

Another cause of RPL is an abnormal female reproductive tract. This can be congenital (i.e., the woman was born with it) or acquired. Congenital anomalies are called *Mullerian anomalies*. The most common Mullerian anomaly that causes RPL is a *septate uterus*, a uterus with an avascular septum dividing the uterine cavity. A woman with a septate uterus generally has no problem getting pregnant but can have RPL due to the embryo implanting on the septum. The septum is fibrous and doesn't have the same healthy blood supply as the normal wall of the uterus. A septate uterus is easily treated surgically with a hysteroscopy. Acquired uterine anomalies are noncongenital and include anything occupying the uterine cavity that prevents an embryo from implanting or growing. Typical acquired uterine anomalies include endometrial polyps, fibroids, or adhesions. Endometrial polyps and fibroids are generally noncancerous growths in the uterine cavity. Intrauterine adhesions are scar tissue that develops in the uterine cavity, usually from a prior uterine procedure. Endometrial polyps, fibroids, and intrauterine adhesions can all be treated surgically with a hysteroscopy.

Thrombophilias are another cause of recurrent pregnancy loss. *Thrombophilia* literally means the "love of blood." Women with these disorders are prone to blood clots, particularly blood clots that block the blood vessels that supply the growing embryo. Because little to no blood supply or nutrients can reach the embryo, the embryo will stop growing. The most common thrombophilias that are tested for with RPL are *antiphospholipid antibody syndrome* (APLS) and lupus anticoagulant. The blood test for APLS is a panel of multiple labs. If you test positive for APLS, the labs will often need to be repeated in twelve weeks to confirm the diagnosis. Once you have been diagnosed with APLS, blood thinners and low-dose aspirin taken throughout the pregnancy increase the chance of a successful pregnancy.

Other causes of RPL include poorly controlled diabetes, hyperprolactinemia, and thyroid disease. These disorders were mentioned in detail in chapter 2. Habits that could potentially lead to pregnancy loss include excessive alcohol intake, excessive caffeine intake, obesity, or use of tobacco or cocaine.[4] It is important to get all medical problems under control first before conceiving.

A thorough evaluation of all possible causes of RPL is critical. A comprehensive assessment of the uterine cavity is essential to evaluate it for congenital or acquired anomalies. We typically check the *karyotypes* (genetic makeup) of the parents to evaluate for balanced translocations. Blood testing for APLS, lupus anticoagulant, diabetes, prolactin, and thyroid disease is generally done. The most frustrating part of RPL is that approximately 50 percent of RPL cases are unexplained.[5] Many patients actually find it difficult to undergo the testing and have all the testing come back normal. The treatment for unexplained RPL is to try to get pregnant after eliminating as many of the possible causes. In many cases of unexplained RPL, empiric (given without clear indication) progesterone and low-dose aspirin are given to prevent pregnancy loss. IVF with PGT-A is a fantastic treatment because we know that we are putting a euploid embryo (an embryo with the correct number of chromosomes or gene regions) into the uterus, so aneuploidy is less likely to be the source of pregnancy loss in this case. It is important to emphasize that, depending on maternal age and parity, the chances of a future successful pregnancy can exceed 50–60 percent in couples with unexplained RPL.[6]

I have been told by women (including my own mother, who lost two children) that the loss of a pregnancy or a child is more emotionally difficult than never conceiving. The unconditional love that a mother has for a child, including her unborn child, is one of the deepest bonds in human existence. Many women with RPL have anxiety and/or depression as a result of their losses. It is crucial that women struggling with RPL see a therapist, counselor, or psychologist. Many can also benefit from support groups, which reinforce that they are not alone.

NOTES

1. Practice Committee of the American Society for Reproductive Medicine, "Definitions of Infertility and Recurrent Pregnancy Loss: A Committee Opinion," *Fertility and Sterility* 99, no. 1 (2013): 63.

2. J. M. Franasiak et al., "The Nature of Aneuploidy with Increasing Age of the Female Partner: A Review of 15,169 Consecutive Trophectoderm Biopsies Evaluated with Comprehensive Chromosomal Screening," *Fertility and Sterility* 101, no. 3 (2014): 656–63.

3. H. Elghezal et al., "Prevalence of Chromosomal Abnormalities in Couples with Recurrent Miscarriage," *Fertility and Sterility* 88, no. 3 (2007): 721–23; F. Kavalier, "Investigation of Recurrent Miscarriages," *British Medical Journal* 331 (2005): 121–22.

4. M. L. Lindbohm, M. Sallmen, and H. Taskinen, "Effects of Exposure to Environmental Tobacco Smoke on Reproductive Health," supplement, *Scandinavian Journal of Work, Environment, and Health* 28, S2 (2002): 84–86; C. Boots and M. D. Stephenson, "Does Obesity Increase the Risk of Miscarriage in Spontaneous Conception: A Systematic Review," *Seminars in Reproductive Medicine* 29, no. 6 (2011): 507–13; R. B. Ness et al., "Cocaine and Tobacco Use and the Risk of Spontaneous Abortion," *New England Journal of Medicine* 340, no. 5 (1999): 333–39; U. Kesmodel et al., "Moderate Alcohol Intake in Pregnancy and the Risk of Spontaneous Abortion," *Alcohol and Alcoholism* 37, no. 1 (2002): 87–92; Practice Committee of the American Society for Reproductive Medicine, "Evaluation and Treatment of Recurrent Pregnancy Loss: A Committee Opinion," *Fertility and Sterility* 98, no. 5 (2012): 1103–11.

5. "Evaluation and Treatment of Recurrent Pregnancy Loss."

6. "Evaluation and Treatment of Recurrent Pregnancy Loss."

Seven

The Psychological Component of Fertility

Women who struggle with infertility, recurrent pregnancy loss, and the need to use third-party reproduction can also struggle with anxiety and/or depression. The desire for a child coupled with the inability to have one would depress anyone. Anxiety and depression can then make getting pregnant in future cycles more difficult; there is a vicious cycle between anxiety, depression, and infertility. Mood disorders and infertility are so delicately intertwined that it becomes difficult to separate them.[1]

Stress related to infertility is probably the greatest contributor to infertility-associated anxiety and depression, and mood disorders are a large component of fertility. We have all heard stories of couples who tried for years to conceive, then conceived once they had adopted a child. Or couples who spent years and a lot of money to conceive their first child but then had an unexpected conception of a second child. While there *are* real, physiological causes of infertility, as described in prior chapters, anxiety and depression can have a negative impact on fertility as well.

Mood disorders know no boundaries, for we are all susceptible to them regardless of culture, religion, sexual orientation, or socioeconomic status. In certain cultures, the woman is blamed for the lack of children even though it is her husband who has the problem. Religion can also play a role. For example, a woman of strict Catholic faith may have to weigh her faith against her desire to have children by utilizing IVF. A career woman who has worked hard to have "everything in life" and has certainly encountered stresses along the way will feel anxious about the failure to conceive since she is accustomed to succeeding when she puts in the effort. Fertility treatments can be expensive. A person paying out of pocket or someone of lower socioeconomic status will certainly feel the stresses of finances more than the person who has insurance coverage or is of higher socioeconomic status. Stress can lead to behaviors like drug and alcohol addiction to ease the anxiety. In all cases, reducing stress is helpful.

Ways to reduce stress include seeing a psychologist, therapist, or counselor. Support groups are incredibly helpful; many women feel alone and isolated, but there are other women going through similar challenges. You can find support groups by asking at your fertility clinic or through RESOLVE (the National Infertility Association), the American Fertility Association, Fertile Hope (the Livestrong Foundation), or numerous online groups. Many women will do well just with therapy and support groups. FertiCalm and FertiStrong are apps you can download to your phone that provide coping mechanisms for dealing with the many situations that can cause stress during the fertility journey. Some patients with severe anxiety and depression may need to see a psychiatrist for medications.

Doing activities that you enjoy can also reduce stress. For instance, some women find moderate exercise, yoga, massages, reading a good book, or meeting up with a friend for lunch very relaxing. A healthy psychological component can truly be beneficial for pregnancy.

NOTES

1. Dorette Noorhasan, "Does Psychiatric Diagnosis Affect Fertility Outcomes?," in *Women's Reproductive Mental Health Across the Lifespan*, ed. D. L. Barnes (Switzerland: Springer International, 2014), 141–58.

Epilogue

I hope you have found this fertility manual helpful. I, too, had fertility problems, which I have detailed in my biography, *Miracle Baby: A Fertility Doctor's Fight for Motherhood.* My husband, who is not in the medical field, read the first draft of this book. He told me that he wished someone had given him this book to read before we did all of our IVF cycles. He had to learn all of it by living through it, which was a scary process for him! Even I struggled with the emotional roller coaster of getting my hopes up just to have them shattered a few weeks later. And I, too, have shed tears of despair so many times that I could have overflowed a river. Happily, the last tears I cried were cried the day my son was born. After many years of struggle, I am now a parent!

Both my husband and I are lucky that I am a fertility physician who comprehends the medical jargon and could explain it to my husband in simpler terms. Many people, perhaps yourself included, are not as lucky. I wrote this book to help you understand the fertility process and to equip you to ask the right questions on your road to parenthood. I truly wish you the best of luck. With all of the options now available for parenthood, there's always hope.

Glossary

Adhesions: Scar tissue.

Aneuploid: A cell that has an abnormal number of chromosomes or gene regions (more or fewer than normal) as compared to a normal cell.

Aneuploidy: An abnormal number of chromosomes or gene regions.

Anovulation: Lack of ovulation.

Anti-Mullerian hormone (AMH): A hormone produced by the granulosa cells of the ovarian follicle. The higher the AMH value, the more suggestive of a higher quantity of remaining eggs.

Antral follicle count (AFC): The number of follicles (sacs of fluids containing eggs) in both ovaries as seen on ultrasound at any given time.

Balanced translocation: Generally, all of the chromosomal material necessary for normal growth and development is present but is not arranged correctly. Typically, a section of one chromosome is attached to another chromosome.

Bicornuate uterus: An abnormal uterine type that a woman can be born with. A bicornuate uterus has two horns and can result in infertility, recurrent pregnancy loss, or preterm delivery.

Blastocyst: The stage of the embryo at which the embryo has a blastocyst cavity, inner cell mass, and trophectoderm.

Blastomere: A cell formed during cell division of an embryo.

Cervix: The opening to the uterus.

Chromosome: The structure in a cell that holds genetic information as DNA (deoxyribonucleic acid).

Clomiphene-resistant PCOS: Failure of a woman with PCOS to ovulate after receiving 150 mg of clomiphene citrate daily for five days per menstrual cycle for at least three cycles.

Cryobank: A facility that uses very low temperatures to freeze and store cells.

Cytomegalovirus (CMV): A common virus. Most people show no signs or symptoms of infection. Occasionally, someone will have "flu-like" symptoms. CMV infection can result in birth defects or loss of a pregnancy when a pregnant woman is exposed to the virus.

Deoxyribonucleic acid (DNA): The material in each cell that encodes our genetic information.

Dilation and curettage (D and C): A procedure involving opening the cervix and removing the contents of the uterus by suction and/or scratching the lining of the uterus.

Dominant follicle: The largest follicle in the ovary, containing the egg that will ovulate.

Ectopic pregnancy: A pregnancy that has implanted outside the uterus, frequently in the fallopian tube.

Embryo: The term given to the early stage of development of a human offspring.

Endometrial biopsy: Taking a small sample of the lining of the uterus.

Endometrial hyperplasia: Abnormal thickening of the lining of the uterus. Can be treated medically, but some cases may require surgical treatment. If left untreated, endometrial hyperplasia can become endometrial cancer.

Endometrial polyp: A growth of the endometrium.

Endometrium: The lining inside the uterine cavity. The embryo will attach to the endometrium at implantation.

Estradiol: A hormonal form of estrogen made by the ovary.

Estrogen: A group of steroid hormones that foster the development and maintenance of female characteristics.

Estrone: A hormonal form of estrogen made by the ovaries and fat cells.

Euploid: A cell or embryo that has the correct number of chromosomes or gene regions.

Fallopian tube: A tubal structure where the sperm and egg unite to form the embryo. The tube is then used to transport the embryo to the uterus.

Fertilization: The union of the egg and sperm.

Fibroids: Growths of the uterine muscular cells.

Follicles: Sacs of fluid containing eggs. Follicles are found in the ovary.

Follicular phase: The first half of the menstrual cycle. It starts with the onset of menses and ends with ovulation. Follicles grow and mature during this phase.

Follicle stimulating hormone (FSH): A hormone released by the pituitary gland or taken as an injection that stimulates the ovaries.

Fresh embryo transfer: Transfer of embryos back to the uterus just a few days following egg retrieval.

Frozen embryo transfer (FET): Transfer of embryos that have been thawed.

Galactorrhea: Milk production from the breast in a woman who is not pregnant or not breastfeeding.

Gestational carrier: A woman who carries a pregnancy for another person. Colloquially called a surrogate.

Human chorionic gonadotropin (hCG): A hormone produced by the placenta during pregnancy, very similar in structure to luteinizing hormone. Hence, hCG can trigger ovulation in a non-pregnant female.

Hydrosalpinx: A dilated fallopian tube.

Hyperprolactinemia: High levels of prolactin hormone in a woman who is not pregnant or breastfeeding. Women with hyperprolactinemia can present with irregular or loss of menstrual cycles, infertility, milky discharge from the breast, and, in more severe cases, frequent headaches and loss of peripheral vision.

Hyperthyroidism: High levels of thyroid hormone. People with hyperthyroidism can present with weight loss, rapid heart rate, increased appetite, nervousness, anxiety, irritability, tremor, sweating, changes in the menstrual cycle, fine and brittle hair, swelling in the neck (growth of the thyroid), fatigue, and/or increased sensitivity to heat.

Hypothyroidism: Low levels of thyroid hormone. People with hypothyroidism can present with fatigue, hair loss, weight gain, increased sensitivity to cold, changes in the menstrual cycle, constipation, swelling in the neck (growth of the thyroid), and/or dry skin.

Hysterosalpingogram (HSG): An X-ray assessment of the uterus and fallopian tubes as dye is injected into the reproductive system.

Hysteroscopy: A procedure in which an endoscope is placed into the cervix and advanced to the uterine cavity. A hysteroscopy can be used for both evaluation and treatment of uterine problems.

Hysterosonogram: An ultrasound evaluation of the uterus as saline is injected into the reproductive system. Also called a saline infusion sonogram (SIS) or sonohysterogram.

Inner cell mass: The cells of the embryo that will become the baby.

Intracervical insemination (ICI): A procedure in which a semen sample is placed on the cervix.

Intracytoplasmic sperm injection (ICSI): The microscopic process of injecting a single sperm into a single egg.

Intrauterine insemination (IUI): A procedure in which a washed semen sample is placed directly into the uterus using a small catheter.

In vitro fertilization (IVF): The process of fertilizing the egg with sperm outside the female reproductive system. It requires the embryologist to have both the eggs and sperm in the lab.

Luteal phase: The second half of the menstrual cycle. The luteal phase starts after ovulation and ends with the onset of the next menses. Progesterone hormone levels are elevated in the luteal phase.

Luteinizing hormone (LH): A hormone released from the pituitary that stimulates the ovaries. LH elevation triggers ovulation.

Midluteal phase: The luteal phase is the second half of the menstrual cycle (from ovulation to the onset of the next menses). The luteal phase typically lasts fourteen days. Seven days into the luteal phase is considered the midluteal phase. The progesterone hormone is elevated in the luteal phase, with its highest value in the middle of the luteal phase.

Morula: The embryonic stage at which the embryo is a solid ball of cells.

Mullerian anomaly: An abnormality in the female reproductive tract that a woman is born with. Common congenital Mullerian anomalies include septate uterus, bicornuate uterus, and unicornuate uterus.

Oligoovulation: Infrequent ovulation (less than 8 times per year).

Oocyte: An egg (the female reproductive cell).

Ovarian hyperstimulation syndrome (OHSS): A medical condition that results from excessive stimulation of the ovaries in response to hormonal medications. Ovaries can get enlarged and painful. Fluid can accumulate in the belly and/or lungs. Sometimes, the fluid needs to be removed. Most cases are mild. A few cases can be severe. In severe cases, there can be electrolyte abnormalities or blood clots in the legs and/or lungs. OHSS is a self-limiting disease, meaning that if there is no fresh embryo transfer, OHSS will resolve with the onset of the menses following egg retrieval.

Ovarian reserve: A general term that describes the quantity and quality of a woman's eggs.

Ovary: A female reproductive organ that produces eggs (female reproductive cells).

Ovum: A mature egg (female reproductive cell) that can be fertilized to form an embryo.

Pituitary: The gland at the base of the brain that makes and releases various hormones.

Polycystic ovarian syndrome: A syndrome in which a woman has two of the following three characteristics, as based on the Rotherdam 2003 criteria, and has been excluded for other diseases: (1) oligoovuation or anovulation (clinically, the woman will have irregular or no menstrual cycles); (2) clinical or laboratory evidence of excess androgens (hormones like testosterone); (3) polycystic ovaries on sonogram.

Preimplantation genetic testing (PGT): The genetic evaluation of an embryo before transferring the embryo back to the uterus. PGT-A involves testing the embryo for aneuploidy—the presence of abnormal number of chromosomes or gene regions. PGT-M involves testing the embryo for monogenic (single-gene) disorders, in which a parent carries a specific gene that they do not want passed down to the next generation.

Progesterone: The hormone released from the corpus luteum (a remnant of the follicle after ovulation). Elevated progesterone indicates recent ovulation.

Prolactin: A hormone made by the pituitary gland. Elevation of this hormone can cause irregular or absent menstrual cycles, infertility, galactorrhea, and, in severe cases, headache and loss of peripheral vision.

Reciprocal in vitro fertilization (IVF): IVF in a female same-sex couple in which the eggs of one female are retrieved and fertilized with donor sperm. The resulting embryo is later transferred to her female partner.

Saline infusion sonogram (SIS): An ultrasound evaluation of the uterus as saline is injected into the reproductive system. Also called a hysterosonogram or sonohysterogram.

Septate uterus: A congenital uterine anomaly in which an avascular septum divides the uterine cavity.

Sonohysterogram: An ultrasound evaluation of the uterus as saline is injected into the reproductive system. Also called a hysterosonogram or saline infusion sonogram (SIS).

Sperm: A male reproductive cell.

Surrogate: A term used colloquially for gestational surrogacy or a gestational carrier, meaning the woman carrying the pregnancy is not biologically related to the pregnancy.

Thrombophilia: A blood-clotting disorder.

Transvaginal oocyte retrieval (TVOR): An ultrasound-guided procedure involving removal of the oocytes (eggs) through a needle inserted in the vagina.

Trophoblast: Another term for trophectoderm. The cells of the embryo that will become the placenta.

Trophectoderm: Another term for trophoblast. The cells of the embryo that will become the placenta.

Tubal ligation: A method of sterilization where the fallopian tubes are bound, transected, or completely removed.

Unicornuate uterus: An abnormal type of uterus a woman can be born with. A woman with an unicornuate uterus has a uterus with one horn and one fallopian tube. These women are at increased risk of infertility, recurrent pregnancy loss, and preterm labor.

Uterus: The organ in the female pelvis that carries a baby for nine months.

Vagina: An elastic, muscular canal that extends from the cervix to the external genitalia.

Vitrification: A method of rapidly freezing cells.

Zona pellucida: The outer layer of the egg, colloquially described as the "eggshell." It is a strong, transparent membrane surrounding the oocyte (egg).

Zygote: A fertilized egg.

Acknowledgments

I would like to thank my patients, who inspire me every day.

My deepest thanks to my husband and best friend, who read the first draft of this book. He has been my biggest supporter and number-one fan.

Susan Hudson, MD, has been one of my dear friends and colleagues for more than a decade. She read the first draft of this book and provided valuable feedback. Thank you, Susan, for your kindness.

Huge props to my parents. They brought me into this world and sacrificed a lot so I could pursue my dreams. I will forever be grateful for their love and support.